YOUR KNOWLEDGE HAS VALUE

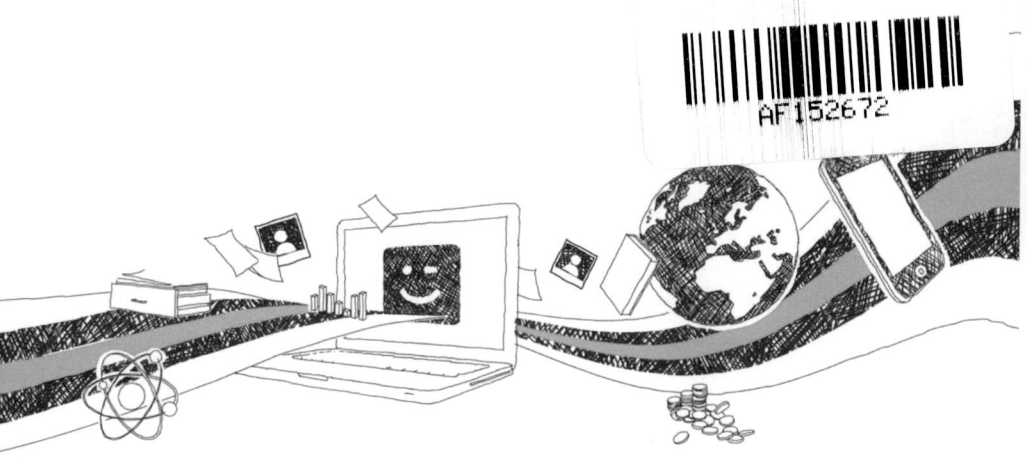
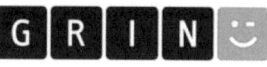

Kirsten Hermes

Keep the Balance right - Ethical issues and the view to quarantine during the SARS outbreak

GRIN Publishing

Bibliographic information published by the German National Library:

The German National Library lists this publication in the National Bibliography; detailed bibliographic data are available on the Internet at http://dnb.dnb.de .

Imprint:

Copyright © 2007 GRIN Verlag GmbH
Print and binding: Books on Demand GmbH, Norderstedt Germany
ISBN: 978-3-640-14981-0

This book at GRIN:

http://www.grin.com/en/e-book/114593/keep-the-balance-right-ethical-issues-and-the-view-to-quarantine-during

GRIN - Your knowledge has value

Since its foundation in 1998, GRIN has specialized in publishing academic texts by students, college teachers and other academics as e-book and printed book. The website www.grin.com is an ideal platform for presenting term papers, final papers, scientific essays, dissertations and specialist books.

Visit us on the internet:

http://www.grin.com/

http://www.facebook.com/grincom

http://www.twitter.com/grin_com

Keep the balance right

-

Ethics and Quarantine

Ethical issues and the view to quarantine during the SARS outbreak

A Summary of research facts

University of Applied Sciences Hamburg
Department Public Health
by Kirsten Hermes
2006

Keep the balance right
Ethical issues and the view to quarantine during the SARS outbreak

Abstract:

Decision making in public health crises is associated with a high potential on ethical conflicts especially in restricting liberty measures such as quarantine. An effective and acceptable public health coping has the dual role of monitoring compliance and providing support to people in quarantine.

The global 2003 nonmedical response to severe acute respiratory syndrome (SARS) and experiences in various states like China, Vietnam, Singapore or Canada with large – scale quarantine, raised ethical questions in seeking the right balance between the tension of protecting the public`s health and human rights and human needs. The loss of liberty, privacy and free movement as well as experienced psychosocial harm like fear, discrimination and stigmatization were discribed as collateral damage but found problematic, also for further successful voluntary compliance.

This paper focusses on both sides and attempts to find recommendations for effective and acceptable use of quarantine in public health policies based on applied ethical values. By analyzing the quarantine experiences there are serious lessons to be prepared for future threats like SARS or SARS - like diseases with pandemic potential.

(177 words)

Key words: quarantine, compliance, ethics in public health emergencies, severe acute respiratory syndrome

Introduction:

Quarantine[1] and isolation is an ancient public health tool to control and prevent the spread of contagious diseases. Already the old testament discribes the sequestering of persons with leprosy as found by *Leviticus*. In the 14th century quarantine was the

---

[1] Quarantine refers to the separation and movement restriction of exposed individuals who are not (yet) ill. Isolation refers to the separation and movement restriction of infected individuals who have a specific infectious transmissible disease.

common practice to control the spread of pneumonic and bubonic plague. The term quarantine derived from the italian *quaranta* meaning 40, was used to prevent disease transmission when officials in Venice forced arriving ships to protect locals from the plague for 40 days [1, 3]. The quarantine practice often has negative connotations, although applied since centuries because of the equation by disease with crime. Quarantined persons, not always separated from ill, were often detained for a long time without regarding their needs and were strongly avoided and stigmatized [1–4]. Until today the implementation evokes a set of emotional reactions such as fear, uncertainty, resentment and associates social isolation and stigmatization as well as doubts in faith of political and social institutions. In a few cases in the past, the power of quarantine was abused to targeted foreigners by stigmatization on social class, race or economic status. For example in the beginning of the 19th century the steerage and third class passengers of ships arriving from Europe to the United States were frequently quarantined and transported to quarantine stations to be examined on contagious diseases while first and second class passengers were briefly examined in their cabins and allowed to disembark or continue their journey [2, 3, 4]

The inconsistent communication to the public by confusion of information were shown in different definitions of "probable cases", "suspect cases" and "cases under investigation" by the WHO and public health officals. Additionally the term "voluntary quarantine" led to public suggestion of discretion and accountability of each person [14].
The contemporary use of quarantine refers to reduce the frequency of transmission by increasing the social distance between exposed and contact persons, which can significantly reduce the spread of an infectious disease. The quarantine strategies can range from active or passive monitoring, short term voluntary home curfew ("sheltering in place"), cancellation of public activities like "snow days" to the point of "cordon sanitaire", which is used in particular crises by erecting a barrier around the affected area [2, 11]. Modern quarantine and contact surveillance is required to preserve the individual liberties based on the *Siracusa Principles*. The application of this intervention must meet the interest of a legitimate objective of general interest by enforcing this public health intervention not arbitrarily, in an unreasonable or discriminatory manner and holding the restriction time-limited and in a review process [21].
This ancient public health intervention tool, also characterized by abuse of power and

discrimination against groups and individuals in the past, but best countermeasures at times with no definitive diagnostic tests, effective vaccines or treatment against the spread of communicable diseases, has been widely used in the first major infectious disease of the 21st century, when the devastating SARS pandemic appeared. Within a short time the novel coronavirus (CoV) had spread rapidly across international borders, so 8445 cases and 774 deaths in 30 countries were finally reported by the World Health Organization (WHO) from Nov 1, 2002 to July 31, 2003 [2, 6]. During the SARS outbreak the data sole for the greater Toronto area was more than 30.000 persons to remain in voluntary quarantine [8].

In autumn 2005 the WHO released an underscored call on planners in influenza and other communicable likely diseases for pandemic preparedness to give attention to ethical issues and applied ethical framework. The emphasis issued such like quarantine concerning to worldwide experience with containment measures when the SARS threat appears [7]. This paper estimates the enforced quarantine during the SARS pandemic and their results due to factors of compliance and attempts to find recommendations for an effective and ethical use of voluntary quarantine in a balanced process.

Background: Quarantine during SARS

China, Hong Kong, Vietnam, Singapore and Canada were hit the hardest caused by the novel corona virus. The median duration time of quarantine during the 2003 pandemic was about 10–12 days, according to the incubation time and time elapsed since exposure. It had been globally imposed to ten thousands of individuals with different sociopolitical and legal regulating systems by home and work containment [6, 7][2]
In Taiwan about 131.000 persons were confined in home quarantine or in "quarantine facilities" [12], Bejing held about 30.000 under similar conditions in quarantine [13]. Utilizable research in studies and experiences of individuals in voluntary quarantine, mainly conducted and published by northamerican especially canadian authors, found

---

[2] The chinese nomenclature did not fit with the established definitions between quarantine and isolation, it was all called "isolation" [8].

inadequate application and inconsistencies concerning ethical questions in view to the collateral damage at the end of the pandemic.

The 2004 *Hawryluck et al.* and *DiGiovanni et al.* studies similarly found except from highly economic impact by the threat itself, the considerable psychological impact resulting from quarantine. Psychologically distress in forms of PTSD (post traumatic stress disorders) and depressive symptoms resulting from fear of illness and death, infecting others, stigmatization and discrimination by avoiding the quarantined persons were found [7-10].

Findings of *DiGiovanni et al.* study on public`s cooperation to quarantine and influencing facts estimated reducing the risk of transmission to another person as the most important reason for complying. The reason due to this considerable principal motivation was found in the civic duty of the protection of the community among health care workers and non health care workers. Moreover, the known fear of penalties by law did not influence the decision to comply to self-quarantine. The most common reasons for noncompliance and demotivating factors were found in the fear of loss of income, the inconsistencies in various application quarantine jurisdictions, inconsistencies in logistical support of quarantined and confused communication3 to the public by government and available media response and communication systems to allow to keep in touch with their families for quarantined individuals [7]. The 2006 published survey by *Blendon et al* estimated the possible use of quarantine in Hong Kong, Taiwan, Singapore and United States. The findings additionaly show a less lower level of compliance and likely change of behaviour particulary in minorities, if people are not concerned about the health threat and don`t have appropriate and accurate information for quarantine preparation [28].

The conclusion of the publications is the simple fact, that quarantine restricts not only individual liberty by limiting freedom of movement and privacy, but also imposes psychological burden, disrupts and isolates individuals from common life and influences compliance to further quarantine by experienced inconsistencies of various supporting issues.

DISCUSSION
Preserving the balance

Quarantine represents a classical conflict that confronts public health in measuring containment strategies in emergencies: the tension between the dual interest of the public in protecting and promoting the citizen`s health and maintaining the individual rights like mobility, privacy and freedom of assembly. Facing the research results about quarantine during the SARS outbreak and the need for an implemented ethical framework in future preparedness plans to minimize the negative adverse affects, there has to be more than the moral obligation for public health decision makers to achieve the greatest good for the greatest number in sense of utilitarianism and moreover deontological ethics. There have been several comments on providing a framework for the analysis of ethical issues in recent years in achieving the balance in serious situations like restricting liberties.

The framework by the research group of the *Joint Centre of Bioethics* Toronto, Canada, takes a step closer into the quarantine practice. The more is the step into an applied ethical action course in such situations. Hence, the following discussion for an applied ethical framework is mainly adapted by their recommendations which were initiated comprehensive applied ethical action on decision making levels and keystones about ethical dimensions in restricting individual liberties in the name of public health [14, 16-22].

Prerequisite for an applicable and operative ethical framework are the 2005 revised *International Health Regulation*s and the *UN Siracusa Principles* [21, 22]. Furthermore, based on the 2003 SARS experience, the research group identified a shared set of substantive ethical issues [15, 17, 20]:

- liberty
- protection of the public from harm
- proportionality
- privacy
- reciprocity
- solidarity and trust

The recommended procedural process requires to be in a reasonable, scientific based manner, which is bound in an open and transparent non-discriminatory discourse.

The first substantive issue of **liberty** means, that the restrictions on individual liberties should be equitable, proportional to necessity and are used as the least restrictive measures, (for example, education, facilitation and discussion), before the full force of state authority can be justified.

The second issue about the **protection of the public from harm** requires the public health authorities to provide serious and immanent reasons for public health restricting measures to encourage the compliance and establish structures to review decisions.

The **proportionality** factor means, when protecting many from harm is ethically necessary, authorities must also protect individuals from needless coercion. Those restrictions of liberty have to be relevant and should not exceed to what is necessary to actual level of risk.

The **privacy** aspect also includes the privacy information and needs acceptance and respect of each person also to prevent further stigmatization.

The **reciprocity** issue requires that the affected society needs in turn to have adequate care (food, medical care, psychosocial care) and implemented mechanisms to avert suffering unfair economic penalties.

Solidarity and trust build the quintessential components in enhancing the whole process as important as **transparency** and can also be seen as a reciproc process in achieving an optimal balance with clear and consistent communication through acountability.

The research group further states three keystones to enhance the communication and clearing the role and application of quarantine [20]:

- the rationale for restrictive measures
- the benefits of compliance and
- the consequences of non-compliance

Some recommendations:

Facing the several distinctive guidelines on the international to local level for quarantine measures there are inconsistencies in various applications of public health law, public health infrastructure and ancillary services or logistical support concerning quarantine, which create confusion to those who want to comply. An important step to a consistent strategy in the operative pandemic plans is the harmonization of several health policies and surveillance systems for future preparedness. According also to the "Measures undertaken by memberstates" by the EU commission in 2003, there are inconsisties in implementation of containment strategies such as quarantine by different or missing guidelines including travel advisories and plans for preventing stigmatization [19, 26]. Hence, the harmonization in public health infrastructure among all levels of government, domestically and internationally coordination is needed.

The SARS epidemic revealed the importance of coping with ethical principles in future preparedness plans to minimize the societal and human costs in public health emergencies when restricting the individual liberties. Decision making in times of scientific uncertainty facing new emerging infectious diseases with pandemic potential need to be founded on widely held ethical values like proportionality, the least restrictive means, transparency and reciprocity to enhance understanding and compliance to restrictive decisions. Achieving the improved balance public health decision makers have to ensure the appropriate support to people affected by quarantine and provide mechanisms to protect stigmatization. However, the ethical implementation of modern quarantine stategies can be resource and labor intensive but most effective, if the intervention is tailored to specific circumstances. Consequently, public health authorities and the public need to be engaged in open and transparent discourses about the ethical dimensions of restrictive measures.

Conclusion:

Enhancing restrictive measures like quarantine and necessary compliance has to compensate individual liberties with protection of public from harm in proportionality and reciprocity. Procedure preparedness guidelines for communicable diseases have to communicate the rationale for restrictive measures, the consequences of non compliance and the benefits of compliance. The process should be held in an open, transparent, fair and non discriminatory process with an implemented back up structure against possible disadvantages and stigmatization on all participating public health action levels.

References:

1. **Slack, P.** (1988): Responses to plague in early modern Europe: the implications of public health. *Social research*, Vol. 55, No. 3, 433-453

2. **Barbera, J., Macintyre, A., Gostin, L. et al** (2001): Large Scale Quarantine Following Biological Terrorsim in the United States – Scientific Examination, Logistics and Legal Limits, and Possible Consequences. *JAMA: The Journal of the American Medical Association,* Vol. 286, No. 21, 2711-2718

3. **Edelson, P. J.** (2003): Quarantine and social Inequity. *JAMA: The Journal of the American Medical Association,* Vol. 290 (21), 2874

4. **Gensini, G.F., Yacoub, M. H., Conti, A. A.,** (2004): The concept of quarantine in history: from plague to SARS. *Journal of Infection,* Vol. 49, 257-261. Available at: http://www.elsevierhealth.com/journals/jinf. Accessed 2005, Nov 5 (this url was not available in 13/04)

5. **Mandavilli, A.** (2003): SARS epidemic unmasks age-old quarantine conundrum. *Nature Medicine,* Vol. 9, No. 5, 487. Available at: http://www.nature.com/naturemedicine. Accessed 2005, Nov 30

6. **World Health Organization (WHO),** (2003): Summary of probable cases with onset of illness from 1 Nov 2002 to 31 Jul 2003. 2003 Sep 26 [cited 2005 Aug 30]. Available at: http://www.who.int/csr/sars/country/table2003_09_23/en/. Accessed 2005,Sep 30

7. **World Health Organization (WHO),** (2005): WHO Checklist for influenza pandemic preparedness planning. Available at: http://www.who.int/csr/resources/publications/influenza/FluCheck6web.pdf. Accessed 2005, Nov 5

8. **Rothstein, M. A., Alcalde, M. G., Elster, N. R. et al.** (2003): Quarantine and Isolation: Lessons learned from SARS, A report to the Centers for Disease Control and Prevention, Institute for Bioethics, Health Policy and Law; University of Louisville School of Medicine

9. **DiGiovanni, C., Conley, J., Chiu et al** (2004): Factors Influencing Compliance with Quarantine in Toronto During the 2003 SARS Outbreak. *Biosecurity and Bioterrorism: Biodefense Strategy, Practice, and Science,* Vol. 2, No. 4, 265-272

10. **Hawryluck L., Gold, W. L., Robinson, S. et al.** (2004): SARS Control and Psychological Effects of Quarantine, Toronto , Canada. *Emerging Infectious Diseases,* No. 7 July 2004, Centers of Disease Control, 1206-1212

11. **Cetron, M., Maloney, S., Koppaka, R. et al** (2004): Isolation and Quarantine: Containment Strategies for SARS 2003. In: Knobler, S., Mahmoud, A., Lemon, S. et al (Edts.), Learning from SARS – Preparing for the next outbreak – Workshop Summary, Forum on Microbial Threats, Board on Global Health, Institute of Medicine of the National Academics, The National Academie Press, Washington D. C., 71-83. Available at: http://www.nap.edu. Accessed 2005, Nov 5

12. **Centers of Disease Control and Prevention** (2003): Use of quarantine to prevent transmission of Severe Acute Respiratory Syndrome – Taiwan 2003. *Morbidity and Mortality Weekly Report (MMWR)*, Centers of Disease Control, 2003; No. 52, 680-683

13. **Centers of Disease Control and Prevention** (2003): Efficiency of quarantine during an epidemic of Severe Acute Respiratory Syndrome – Bejing, China,2003. *Morbidity and Mortality Weekly Report (MMWR)*, Centers of Disease Control, 2003, No. 52, 1037-1040

14. **Campbell, A.** (2005): The SARS commission second interim report: SARS and Public Health legislation, Ontario, 2005, Apr. 5. Available at: http://www.sarscommission.ca/report/Interim_Report_2.pdf. Accessed 2005, Nov 5, (this url was not available in 13/04)

15. **Singer, P. A., Benatar, S. R., Bernstein, M. et al.** (2003): Ethics and SARS: Learning Lessons from the Toronto Experience, A Report by a working group of the University of Toronto Joint Centre for Bioethics. Available at: http://www.yorku.ca/igreene/sars.html. Accessed 2005, Nov 16.

16. **Mill J.S.,** (1859): On Liberty in: The Philosophy of John Stuart Mill. In: Cohen M., 1961, (Edt.) New York, NY, Modern Library, 185-319

17. **Upshur, R. E. G.** (2002): Principles for the Justification of Public Health Intervention; *Canadian Journal of Public Health*, March-April 2002, Vol. 93 (2), 101-103

18. **Gostin, L. O., Bayer, R., Fairchild, A. L.,** (2003): Ethical and legal challenges posed by severe acute respiratory syndrome. *JAMA: The Journal of the American Medical Association,* Dec. 24/31, Vol. 290 (24), 3229-3237

19. **European Commission SANCO – Public Health Directorate G4 Unit – Communicable, Rare and Emerging Diseases,** 2003: Measures undertaken by member states and accession countries to control the outbreak of SARS. May 28, 2003. Available at: http://europa.eu.int/comm/health/ph_threats/com/sars/sars_measures_en.pdf. Accessed Jan 25, 2006 , The new adress since 2008 of the European Commission is http://ec.europa.eu/

20. **University of Toronto Joint Centre for Bioethics Pandemic Influenza Working Group,** (2005): Stand on gard for thee; Ethical considerations in preparedness planning for pandemic influenza. Available at: http://www.utoronto.ca/jcb/home/documents/pandemic.pdf. Accessed 2006, Jan. 25. (this url was not available in 13/04)

21. **United Nations,** (1984): The Siracusa Principles on the limitation and derogation provisions in the International Convenant on Civil and Political Rights. Available at:http://www.article23.org.hk/english/research/ICCPR.doc+siracusa+principles&hl=en. Accessed 2005, Dec. 13. (this url was not available in 13/04)

22. **World Health Organization (WHO)**, (2005): International Health Regulations, revised April 2005. Available at: http://www.who.int/csr/ihr/current/en/index.html. Accessed 2006, 25 Jan

23. **Kass, N. E.** (2001): An Ethics Framework for Public Health, *American Journal of Public Health*, November 2001, Vl. 91, (11), 1776-1781

24. **Smith, C. B., Battin, M. P., Jacobson, J. A. et al.** (2004): Are there characteristics of infectious diseases that raise special ethical issues?, Discussion paper at the 2003 American Society for Bioethics and Humanities Conference, "Bioethics across Borders", *Developing World Bioethics*, Vol. 4, (1). Available at: http://sitemaker.umich.edu/hpsa/files/smith_et_al.pdf. Accessed 2005, Nov. 30

25. **Coker, R.** (2000): Tuberculosis, non – compliance and detention for the public health. *Journal of Medical Ethics*, Vol. 26, 147-159

26. **Kassen, A.** (2004): International SARS Control: Analysis of European and non – european public health policies, Master Thesis, University of Applied Sciences Hamburg (HAW). Available at: http://www.haw-hamburg.de/bib/diplom/2004/bergedorf/Master/ges_y-67.pdf. Accessed 2005, Nov 5. (this url was not available in 13/04)

27. **Plough, A., Warner, J. E., Loehr, M.** (2004): Isolation and Quarantine: Surviving a Lethal Outbreak; Northwest Public Health, University of Washington School of Public Health. Available at: http://www.nwcphp.org/nph. Accessed 2005, Sep 30. (this url was not available in 13/04)

28. **Blendon, R. J., DesRoches, C. M., Cetron, M. S. et al** (2006): Attitudes toward the use of quarantine in a public health emergency in four countries, The experiences of Hong Kong, Singapore, Taiwan, and the United States are instructive in assessing national responses to disease threats. Datawatch: Quarantine 24 January 2006, Available at: http://content.healthaffairs.org/cgi/content/full/hltfaff.25.w15/DC1. Accessed 2006, Feb. 02, (this url was not available in 13/04)